NURSE PRACTITIONER SCHOOL AND BEYOND

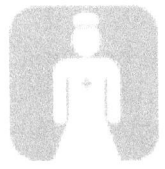

TIPS FOR THE STUDENT NURSE PRACTITIONER

Nachole Johnson

Copyright 2016 Nachole Johnson and ReNursing Publishing Company.
ALL RIGHTS RESERVED.

ISBN: 1539427005

ISBN-13: 978-1539427001

Disclaimer

Although the author and publisher have made every effort to ensure the information provided in this book were correct at press time, the author and publisher do not assume and hereby disclaim any liability to any party for any loss, damage, or disruption caused by errors or omissions, whether such errors or omissions result from negligence, accident, or any other cause.
This book is not intended as the substitute for the legal advice or consultation of attorneys. The reader should regularly consult an attorney in matters relating to his/her business that may require legal advisement.

All rights are reserved. No part of this publication may be reproduced, distributed, more transmitted in any form or by any means, including photocopying, recording, or other electronic or means, including photocopying, recording, or any other electronic or mechanical methods, without the prior written permission of the publisher, except in no commercial use permitted uses permitted by copyright law.

TABLE OF CONTENTS

Why I Wrote This Book

Chapter 1 The NP Scope and Specialties
  Definition of an NP
  Overview of NP Specialties
    Family Nurse Practitioner (FNP)
    Adult Gerontology Acute Care (AGACNP)
    Adult Gerontology Primary Care (AGPCNP)
    Neonatal NP (NNP)
    Pediatric Nurse Practitioner Acute Care (CPNP-AC)
    Pediatric Nurse Practitioner Primary Care (CPNP-PC)
    Women's Health NP (WHNP)
    Psychiatric- Mental Health NP (PMHNP)

Chapter 2 How to Choose an NP Specialty

Chapter 3 Getting into School

Chapter 4 Juggling Work, School and Family
  Managing Work, School and Family
  Managing Your Money While in School

Chapter 5 Study Tips
  Group study
  Studying on Your Own
  Learning Styles

Chapter 6 Clinical Pearls

Chapter 7 Preparing for the Certification Exam
  Nurse Practitioner Certification Boards
  Which Certification Board Should You Take?
  How I Studied for My Certification Exam
  Sample Study Calendar
  Nurse Practitioner Certification Boards Contact Information

Chapter 8 Landing Your First Job
A word on resumes…
5 Tips to Maximize Your Job Hunting Experience
The Interview
- Tips for Acing Your Interview
- Practice Interviewing
- Be Prepared for Odd Questions
- Research the Company
- Be on Time
- Follow-up with a Thank You Note
Questions You Need to Ask During an Interview
Questions You Will Probably be Asked During an Interview
I was offered a job, now what?

Chapter 9 Life After School
Prescriptive Authority as an NP
- NPI number
- Prescriptive Authority
- Collaboration Agreement
- DEA number
Classification of Controlled Substances
Prescription Writing
What Exactly do I Need to Keep up With as an NP?
An NP, by any Other Name
How Do I Sign My Name Now That I'm an NP?

One Last Thing

About the Author

Other Books By Nachole Johnson

Why I Wrote This Book

After graduating from NP school in 2013, I realized I still had many unanswered questions that were not answered in my program. After speaking to many of my classmates, I realized they had the same problem – unanswered questions. Going to NP school was the best thing I could have done for my career at the time. So far, I've enjoyed my chosen career. But I would like to help others who may have questions before choosing this route.

The process of applying, getting through school, and passing my certification exam taught me many lessons I would like to pass along to other prospective NP students. Throughout the process, I had many questions like, "What do I do next?"

In speaking to other colleagues, I found that many NP programs are severely lacking when it comes to important things an NP needs to know like billing and coding, how to find your first job, how to negotiate, things to expect in a contract, etc. My program briefly went over those subjects or some of them, not at all! There were many other unanswered questions like "What types of numbers do I need as an NP (license,

NPI, DEA, etc.) and most importantly, how do I get them?"

I wish I had a book like this one before I applied to NP school. The information would have given me a head start on what to expect in my future career. I believe it is important that schools teach us the basic clinical skills to thrive as an NP but also include business skills as well. We are no longer wage earners who do not generate directly generate revenue. As providers who bill for valuable services, we are moneymakers to those who employ us. NPs need to learn their value in their new role.

It is a very good time to become an NP. Did you know that the *U.S. News and World Report has ranked* the NP profession as one of the top ten best jobs in America and number five in Healthcare jobs? The number of NPs is also on the rise, The United States Bureau of Labor Statistics projects a 31% growth rate for the profession, and there are already more than 222,000 licensed NPs in the United States.

I wrote this book for those wanting to become an NP, student NPs, and those still lost in their first year of practice. I made many mistakes in my first couple of years of an NP, and I want to help others avoid the same ones I made. If this book just offers guidance to one person contemplating the NP profession, then I've done my job.

Chapter 1
The NP Scope and Specialties

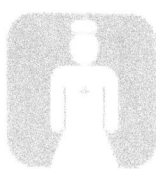

I'm sure if you're reading this book, you already know what a Nurse Practitioner (NP) is. If you are considering the profession, and you don't quite know the role of an NP, this book will help clarify any confusion you may have.

Definition of an NP

An NP, by definition, is a registered nurse who is prepared through advanced training beyond the undergraduate level, to provide a range of health services, including diagnosis and treatment of a wide variety of medical conditions. Furthermore, an NP has earned a license to practice within their specialty in accordance with the state law in which they reside.

Through that additional education and training, comes great responsibility. Often, NPs manage and treat the same conditions as our physician counterparts. Some states have already recognized that we are formidable as primary care providers. There have been studies[1] conducted that compare the outcomes of NPs and MDs, and the results are not statistically significant. That means NPs are competent to treat and manage patients in the many settings where we work. *NPs are legally able to practice with full-authority (without physician involvement) in 21 states and The District of Columbia.[2]

Nurses should choose the NP specialty they want to pursue. Depending on state regulations, certain specialties are more limited in their scope of practice. Additional training in another NP specialty is required to expand the scope of practice. NPs are trained in mostly primary care specialties, and each NP specialty has its special role in healthcare.

Overview of NP Specialties

Here are the NP specialties you can choose to pursue in school.

Family Nurse Practitioner (FNP)

An FNP can see ages from infancy to adulthood. FNPs offer preventative health services, education and disease management. FNPs usually work in outpatient Primary care clinics, but can be found in many other sub-specialties such as Urgent Care, emergency rooms, and rural health clinics.

Adult Gerontology Acute Care (AGACNP)

This specialty is the new designation for the former Acute Care NP. Adult Gerontology Acute Care NPs manage the care of acutely ill adults and seniors, both in the hospital and in specialty clinics. These NPs are trained to manage complex issues and prevent complications. You can find these NPs in acute care and hospital settings such as the MICU, SICU, trauma units and highly specialized outpatient clinics.

Adult Gerontology Primary Care (AGPCNP)

The Adult-Gerontology Primary Care designation was once known as Adult NP. The Adult-Gerontology Primary Care NP can see patients age 13 throughout the senior years. Adult Gerontology NPs work in both inpatient and outpatient settings in a variety of sub-specialties such as internal medicine, prisons, and rehabilitation centers.

Neonatal NP (NNP)

Neonatal NPs deliver care to pre-term and full-term infants, including those with life-threatening conditions and chronic illness. They often time attend high-risk births and are trained in neonatal resuscitation. They receive advanced training to take care of such a fragile and specific population. You will find Neonatal NPs working in newborn nurseries (Level I), Intermediate care nurseries (Level II), and Neonatal intensive care nurseries (Level III).

Pediatric Nurse Practitioner Acute Care (CPNP-AC)

These NPs focus on the acutely ill pediatric population. They can be found working in intensive care units, emergency rooms, and subspecialty clinics. These NPs can also be found in the many children's urgent care centers popping up. Like CPNP-PCs, CPNP-ACs can care for infants, children, adolescents, and young adults.

Pediatric Nurse Practitioner Primary Care (CPNP-PC)

PNP-PCs take care of the primary care needs of children from birth up to young adulthood, mainly in outpatient, non-acute clinics. The focus of their care is on well childcare, prevention, and management of common pediatric acute illnesses and chronic conditions. They can practice in a variety of setting including; but not limited to school-based clinics, private practice, and subspecialty clinics.

Women's Health NP (WHNP)

A women's health NP delivers primary health care to women from adolescent to childbearing and advanced age. They also manage normal and high-risk prenatal care, family planning, fertility, uro-gynecology, and well-woman care. They serve in infertility clinics, women's clinics, and family practice clinics.

Psychiatric- Mental Health NP (PMHNP)

PMHNPs care for the mental health needs of both children and adults. They can assess, diagnose, and treat individuals with mental health disorders. They can be found working in outpatient clinics, hospitals, community centers, and even their private practice. PMHNPs are in high demand because the United States has so few of them. [3]

Chapter 2
How to Choose an NP Specialty

Before you even consider continuing your education, you need to decide why you want to be an NP and what type of NP you want to be. If you do not like nursing, becoming an NP does not guarantee you will like it any better. Generally, NPs function like MDs in settings where everyone is collegial and respects your title as an APRN (Advanced Practice Registered Nurse). If you find yourself in the wrong job setting, you could be treated like a glorified nurse and question why you even went for more education in the first place. This is why it is so important for you to be cautious before you consider the NP profession and before you devote so much time and money toward that goal.

There are many NP specialties, but only a limited number of *certifications* you can pursue based on the population focus you study in school (Neonatal, Pediatric Primary, Pediatric Acute, Women's Health, Family, Adult Geriatric Primary, Adult Geriatric Acute, Psych). NP training is different than Physician's

Assistant or medical training. Our training is focused on a specific population. Medical model students (including MDs and PAs) are trained in all specialties while in school. They complete their generalist training before heading to internships or residencies to specialize.

You should decide which route to pursue in school so you do not feel pigeonholed in your career later. As an example, I had extensive experience in the intensive care unit as an RN, but choose to pursue FNP certification. I believed it would be more marketable than ACNP. After I graduated, I had a hard time finding a job because my RN background did not match my NP certification (more on this later). I soon realized that my ACNP colleagues had an easier time finding jobs.

Look at where you're working now and ask yourself if you would like to stay in that setting as an NP. Remember, your role as an NP differs from an RN because you will be a provider and not take orders from anyone. You will be the one giving orders. If you don't see yourself in a provider role in the setting you are in now, then another specialty may be better suited for you.

I want to touch on a subject that some consider sensitive – the experience required before applying to school. Many nurses say going straight to NP school after your first year of nursing is just fine. Others insist that more time as a nurse is beneficial. I believe more nursing experience is valuable to program applicants and future NPs. I'll tell you why.

The role of a nurse and an NP seldom cross because their functions are so different. I know you're saying, "Wait, what? You just said more nursing experience is beneficial for NP applicants and future NPs." Yes, I did. Longer nursing experience gives exposure you cannot get if you go to graduate school after only one year at the bedside. My many years of nursing experience have often helped me think more critically. I have also seen many medical conditions while working in various settings that still help me today as a practicing NP.

You may take my advice with a grain of salt, but I believe the more nursing experience you have, the better NP you will be.

You should also take into consideration the number of clinical hours NPs get while in school. We usually only receive 600-700 hours for the program. The reason we have so little clinical time as NPs is because schools assume we have gleaned a lot of basic knowledge through our experience as a nurse. If you don't have that basic foundation as an expert nurse, how effective are you going to be as a practicing NP? One year of experience cannot make anyone an expert nurse because they have not yet been exposed to varied situations.

You have many NP certifications to choose for school, but you must be sure you find the right fit for you and your goals. You do have the possibility of dual certification, but that means going to school longer and maintaining the requirements for both certifications.

Where you live should also play a role in the certification you pursue because your certification may make it more difficult to find a job in your area. I suggest you take a look at local job boards and speak to other nurse practitioners in your area to ask about the climate for a particular certification. If you're open to moving to another area after graduation, this isn't a major problem. If you're established and/or have a family and need to stay in the same area, it's best if you do your research before you go to school.

Remember how I was telling you earlier that I had a hard time finding a job after graduation because my RN experience didn't match my NP education? This is a classic example of why you should test the waters to see what certifications are in demand in your area.

Apparently the ACNP (Acute Care NP, now retired) designation seems to be a hot commodity in my area. I chose the FNP route because I didn't want to work in the hospital. However, I didn't know that the certification would keep me from specializing in areas like outpatient pulmonology, cardiology, or infectious disease. That does not mean FNPs can't work in those areas in another city, but in my area I choose the wrong population focus for the jobs I wanted after graduation.

Another thing to consider is that many people (including doctors, recruiters, and patients) don't know the full capability of NPs. They don't realize what we can do and don't understand the scope of the different population focuses. For example, I was trained as an FNP who can see patients ages birth to 100, but couldn't land a job working with pediatric patients. Why? Everyone wanted me to have pediatric experience as an RN even though NPs and RN have different roles when working with children.

So here I was, a critical care RN with an FNP degree, but I couldn't find a job in pediatrics or a specialty other than family medicine. I know what you're thinking, "Why did you go for FNP if you didn't want to work in a family medicine clinic?" For starters, family medicine does not pay well. Second, during my clinical rotations, I decided I didn't like my family medicine or even internal medicine rotations as much as I thought I would.

I've since found a specialty I'm happy with where my ACNP colleagues can't work because they don't have pediatric training in school. I don't see pediatric patients every day in my practice, but my training in this specialization made me marketable for the position.

Chapter 3
Getting into School

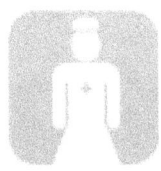

After you figure out what population focus you want to study, the next step is finding a school that supports your future goal. Not all NP schools have every NP certification under one roof (which is another way our education differs from MDs and PAs), but our tuition is much lower in many cases. NP education costs vary across the board. When looking into programs, consider the cost of tuition you'd be paying. If you have to take out loans for a program make sure you choose a specialty or live in a geographic location that will pay you enough to repay it comfortably. In 2016, no NP should make less than $100k per year. Period.

NP education can be completed on campus, online, or in a hybrid setting. I suggest attending a brick and mortar hybrid program because it hurts our reputation as a profession when we complete our degrees completely online. Remember, many employers look at the school where you graduated to see if it is reputable, and most online-only programs don't fit that category, especially if it's your first master's degree and not a post-master program. Be very cautious about attending an online school for your NP degree.

Another thing that sets NP education apart from other medical training is our clinical education. Most NP schools require students to find their own clinical preceptors, but MDs and PAs have their rotations set-up for them. A few schools locate clinical sites for their students, and if you find one, that is a good sign. I am not saying schools that do not provide clinical sites or preceptors are awful. I'm just saying it's rare to find a school that does.

Take into consideration the pass/fail rates for the particular program you want to attend. The passing rate of recent graduates on their national certification exam reveals much about the quality of training they have received. Interview the program director of each program you are considering and ask about pass/fail rates, prospective jobs you can expect after graduation, and what you can do to become more competitive as an applicant.

If you find people who attend that school or have attended the school for their NP degree, question them too. You can learn so much from just doing simple interviews with people who have an insider's perspective.

Finally, you need to decide whether or not you want a master's degree (MSN) or a doctorate (DNP). The DNP is not required to become a practicing NP, but it is considered the terminal degree for the profession. The length of each program varies between 3-5 years depending on if you go full or part-time, MSN or DNP.

With all this being said, you might wonder what the differences are between a MSN NP and a DNP NP. The MSN NP can do everything the DNP NP can do, with very little to no pay increase in many cases. The DNP, although a clinical doctoral degree, is becoming more popular in the academic setting. In the future, those pursuing an academic career may be required to have earned a DNP for most institutions.

To get into school, you must have everything in a basic application packet: application, application fee, references, transcripts, an essay, a CV, and letters of recommendation (may sometimes be the same as references depending on the program). When you find a few schools that interest you, look at their admission requirements and start gathering the items needed. Each school has a deadline when the application packet must be submitted, so it's best to have your materials and references ready when the time comes.

Regarding references, schools have different requirements but many require three; one from your current manager, one from a previous instructor, and one from a professional (it looks good having one from an MD with whom you have worked).

Start working on your application packet months in advance, and keep everything in a safe place. Some schools are notorious for losing things, so keep additional copies of important documents that would take time to replace if you needed them in a hurry.

It's always a good idea to submit your application well in advance of the deadline in case some requirements are misplaced at the school or you lose track of the deadline. Call the school to confirm that they have everything needed for your application. Do this a few weeks before the deadline to be on the safe side.

If the school verifies that your packet is complete, it's just a waiting game for notification of an interview or a letter stating that you didn't get into the program. After your packet submission call the school and speak with an advisor for your program and ask when you should hear back about an acceptance or declination into the program.

At this point, just cross your fingers and wait!

If for some unfortunate reason you don't get in the program of your choice, check with an advisor to see if you can take some prerequisite classes to lighten your course load if you get in the next year. Most NP schools will allow anyone take the three P's (pathophysiology, pharmacology and physical assessment) before they are accepted into a program. In fact, I recommend that all nurses considering graduate education should take a few classes here and there to lighten your course load. You'll be happy you did when your classmates are swamped with 9 credit hours in a semester but you only have 3 or 6 to study.

Chapter 4
Juggling Work, School and Family

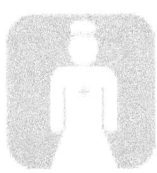

Yay! You got the call, and you were accepted into an NP program. What do you do next?

Now is the time to prepare for the next few years of your life as a graduate student. Like many nurses who pursue NP school, you're probably still working and will still have to work while you go through the program.

If you're one of the many who still have to work during the program, try to prepare yourself financially. Having adequate savings before you start school would be the ideal situation. You can get though most of the program with little difficulty if you have extra money in the bank and aren't stressed over paying the bills.

If you took prerequisites before entering the program, you'll be able to work more and study more when you classmates are stressing about balancing the demands of school and work.

Managing Work, School and Family

You can work while attending school if you work the traditional three 12's per week until your clinicals start. When clinicals start, you will have to reduce your hours, especially if you chose a primary care population focus that mainly works Monday through Friday (Family, pediatric, Women's health, etc.). In these cases, your clinical hours will be based on your preceptors work schedule.

If you have a family at home, you must make it clear to them that you need time alone to study. I know it is hard, but many other working parents have done it. Use some creative techniques during this time like cooking with a crockpot to speed up meal prep time, studying while taking breaks at work, and playing "school" with the younger kids so they can study while you study.

Part of going to graduate school while still working is jugging everything that comes along with it. From the work standpoint, your job needs to be flexible so you can go to class and finish assignments before their due date. An option to consider is going per-diem at work instead of staying full-time. I did so during my clinical rotation just so I could have additional flexibility. I lost my most of my benefits from work (but my medical insurance at school was so much better!), but was able to work as little or as much as I wanted during this time. If you have a family and lots of family events, you may have to miss them or study while you are at your child's events. NP school is a sacrifice that will pay off in the long run.

Managing Your Money While in School

Your finances during school depend on many factors: whether you're married or single, have kids, go to a private school or state school, etc. Whatever your situation, the best bet for someone pursuing NP school is to save as much money as possible beforehand so you won't have to stress out about bills when you should be studying.

Put yourself in the best financial shape as possible before you start because you may have to take days off during your clinical rotations to meet your hours. Unless you work a Baylor-type schedule (Weekends-only) you will need to use some of your PTO to meet your clinical hours, especially in your final semester.

Plan to have at least six months worth of living expenses saved and PTO in your bank at work before you start school.

Your employer may provide tuition-reimbursement to help ease your financial burden during school. I wasn't able to get tuition assistance since I didn't work full-time during school. I had no choice but to work.

Juggling didactic, clinicals, and work is not an easy feat, but it can be done. Every NP that you meet had to make significant sacrifices and adjustments to complete their program and gain certification in their specialization. You have that same potential if you have the desire to reach this goal.

Chapter 5
Study Tips

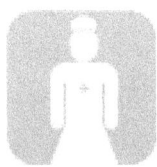

I'm sure your grades were stellar, and that's one of the reasons you were able to get into NP school, but the study methods you used in undergrad may not work in graduate school.

The sheer volume of information you have to digest in graduate school in such as short time will cause some adjustment in the way you study from now on. I never really thought nursing school was hard, but maybe this was because I started as a nurse's aide and LPN before I became an RN.

Because I had previous experience in the nursing field, I was able to build on this knowledge with each level of nursing I pursued. The previous experience did help in my new role of NP student and still helps me today as a practicing NP.

Group study

In grad school, I had to learn to skim while reading and highlighting the most important aspects of a passage. I also had to learn to study with others to gain a better understanding of topics and for the repetition that comes with working in a group.

I know many people may prefer to study on their own and not others, but group study has benefits. Here are three reasons I gravitated to group study while in NP school; 1) It helped me cement concepts already familiar to me, 2) It helped me gain a better understanding of concepts when I was unsure. 3) Believe it or not, I focused better with a study group. We planned on working on a certain subject and stuck to it during our session.

Keeping your group on the smaller side (4-5) makes things easier so no one gets lost in the group during discussion, and the small size avoids erroneous side conversations during study time.

Studying on Your Own

If you plan to study alone, you need to set a study schedule for yourself. When you do this you stay on track, and a balanced schedule gives you enough time to cover all your lecture topics. Try your best to stick to your study schedule. You'll find that with a schedule you'll become more productive.

When you schedule your study time, also include break times so you can stay productive during your study session. I found I could only focus for 45 minutes at a time before my mind started to drift. I started setting a timer for 45 minutes when I began studying and taking a 15-minute break for every one-hour study session. The breaks helped me re-focus, and I used that time to stretch, take a bathroom break, and get a snack.

Consider using flash cards to supplement your study. Flash cards were a main staple of my solo study time. The benefits of using flash cards were threefold for me 1) Visualization by writing the words on the flash card, 2) repetition of the material, and 3) The ability to study anywhere I was without lugging around lots of folders.

Keep your study space in a neutral place if you are studying with a group or alone, making sure it's a quiet place without distractions.

What type of learner are you? Make the most of your learning style while you are in grad school, because you'll need it! Here is the breakdown of the four different learning styles and study tips for each one. Most people don't fit in just one category and are a mix of learning types. Figure out how you study best and use these tips to maximize your study time in school.

Learning Styles [4]

Kinetic: This learner learns best by hands on experience. They are considered "doers" and process more information if they are actively participating.

Characteristics:

- Good with their hands
- Good at remembering things
- Become fidgety when sitting for a long time
- Tend to have poor handwriting or spelling

Study Tips for Kinetic learners:

- Study in short blocks of time and take breaks
- Study in groups
- Use flash cards

Auditory: Auditory learners learn best while actively listening. This group of learners does not take many notes during class because they can learn by listening intently. They also like to talk a lot.

Characteristics:
- Have great memories for conversations and music
- Enjoy discussions, debates, and talking to others
- Prefer oral presentations over written reports
- May read slowly

Study Tips for Auditory Learners

- Ask questions during lecture
- Watch videos (YouTube, anyone?)
- Use Mnemonics
- Repeat information out loud

Visual: These types of learners learn best through what they see.

Characteristics:

- Loves pictures and diagrams
- Create pictures in their mind when reading
- Like bright colors
- May be slow to process a speech or lecture

Study Tips:

- Draw diagrams
- Watch videos
- Use highlighters
- Use flash cards

Read & Write learners: These learners are good traditional studiers, the ones who read textbooks and take notes. They study best by reading their notes or copying them out.

Characteristics:

- Enjoy reading
- Would rather read by themselves rather than someone reading to them
- Often take verbatim or exhaustive notes in class
- Work best in the quiet
- Look up definitions in the dictionary if they come across a word they don't know

Study Tips for Read & Write Learners:

- Take lots of notes
- Rewrite the notes
- Use bullet point lists
- Use handouts given to you in school

Chapter 6
Clinical Pearls

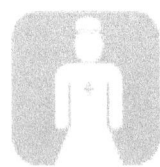

Studying for didactic classes and managing your clinical rotations is a difficult adjustment, but I learned some tips that helped me tremendously during my rotations.

- Contact your preceptor immediately to schedule your clinical rotations well in advance; weeks, sometimes months in advance.

- If you need to do something for your first day of clinicals like get an ID badge or information for the EMR, do so well in advance of your first day.

- Show up about 15 minutes early to your clinical site to ensure you're not late.

- Wear comfortable shoes because you are likely to be on your feet all day.

- Bring your lunch and some snacks to eat on the go during the day. You may not be able to leave the clinical site for lunch.

- Prep your NP bag the night before, and pack it with items such as your stethoscope, clinical reference guides, pens, and a notebook.

- Find your preceptors early in the school year. The best preceptors are often booked many months in advance.

- Use word-of- mouth with your nursing network to find preceptors, including the local NP associations.

- Ask classmates if they recommend a preceptor you can work with during clinicals.

- Try to do clinicals at least two days per week so you don't forget what you learned from week to week. This can easily happen if you only do them once per week.

- Prepare for each clinical rotation by reading on the most common diagnoses seen in that specific setting and identify some differentials beforehand.

- Read about the most common meds and dosages used in your particular clinical setting.

- Download apps that could be useful during your rotation (Epocrates, Medscape, Up-to-Date, etc.)

- "I don't know" is not an acceptable answer to a question. Make sure you know how to find the answer if you don't know it (see above tip)

- Keep a notebook handy during your rotation so you can take notes from each of your preceptors.

- Ask your preceptor if you can take home a blank paper copy of the charting (if they still use paper) so you will know how to correctly document each case.

- Keep your own personal example of a SOAP note handy for reference.

- If they have an EMR (electronic medical records), ask if you can have temporary access to learn how to chart on the system.

- Ask your preceptor for copies of resources they use in clinical practice like cheat sheets for procedures they perform daily.

- Be nice to the front office. They are grading you too (indirectly)!

- Ask your preceptors questions while you can. You are there to learn.

- Be prepared to answer questions from your preceptor. They are trying to judge your incoming knowledge base.

- Know how to competently perform a History and Physical (H&P) before your first clinical day.

- Ask if you can perform specific procedures that you have learned in school.

- Try to see as many patients as you can during clinicals. You are going to be on your own sooner than you think!

- Log your clinical hours into your school's software regularly and consistently. You don't want to get behind on this. You also don't want to be short on hours and not be able to graduate.

- After clinicals, read and research about any interesting case you saw that day.

- Read up on *all* your cases for the day, especially if you struggled with treating.

- Don't just shadow your preceptor. Jump in and see patients on your own when they let you.

- Ask your preceptor if they know other preceptors with whom you could complete your other clinical rotations.

- Ask your preceptor about any open positions in their company or if they have any colleagues who are hiring.

Chapter 7
Preparing for the Certification Exam

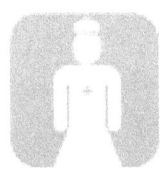

During your last semester of school, you should start preparing for your national certification exam. For your initial certification, the board testing you with will need your transcripts and a validation form from your school confirming that you have completed the education requirements for the specific specialty.

The board with which you certify depends on what your population focus was in school and sometimes on your preference.

Refer to the table on the next page to determine the proper board for your certification.

Nurse Practitioner Certification Boards

Nurse Practitioner Certification	Certifying Board
Adult-Gerontology Acute Care (AGACNP)	ANCC
Adult-Gerontology Primary Care (AGPCNP)	ANCC, AANP
Family (FNP)	ANCC, AANP
Neonatal (NNP-BC)	NCC
Pediatric Acute Care (CPNP-AC)	ANCC, PNCB
Pediatric Primary Care (CPNP-PC)	ANCC, PNCB
Psychiatric Mental Health (PMHNP)	ANCC
Women's Health (WHNP)	NCC

Key: ANCC-*American Nurses Credentialing Center*, AANP- *American Academy of Nurse Practitioners*, NCC-*National Certification Corporation*, PNCB-*Pediatric Nursing Certification Board*

Which Certification Board Should You Take?

If you haven't already noticed, some NP specialties can obtain their board certification through more than one certification board. It is not necessary to be board certified by both centers. One is enough to make you an official NP.

Some people have no choice and must certify with a specific board like Neonatal, Women's Health, and Psychiatric Mental Health. For the other certifications, you have a choice depending on your preference. The different board certifications have different test formats and designations once you pass. For example, if I had taken the AANP board exam instead of the ANCC exam my title would be Nachole Johnson, MSN, FNP-C instead of Nachole Johnson, MSN, FNP-BC.

I had friends who took their boards through AANP because they heard that the ANCC exam had more areas covered than just clinical focus (true). Others said one exam seemed like it would be harder than the other. I personally took the ANCC exam simply because I wanted "BC" behind my name instead of "C." I found the ANCC exam to be straightforward. There wasn't a question presented about which I didn't at least know a little.

I'm letting you in on my study method so maybe it will help you be successful with your exam.

How I Studied for My Certification Exam

You can choose a variety of ways to study for your certification boards, so you must determine which works best for you. I used a variety of methods to study for my exam. I was successful with passing my exam and actually found it rather easy.

I purchased a certification review book, read it, and went over the practice questions and rationales multiple times. As a matter of fact, during my last semester of school, I used the review book to study for my school courses. I didn't use multiple review books, just two.

Some prefer to use books written by Fitzgerald, Hollier, or Leik, but it really doesn't matter. You do need to practice the questions and read rationales to gain a greater understanding of the content.

Just in case you wanted to know, I used a Fitzgerald review book. I found it to be the most straightforward book of those available. The only other book I used was the *ANCC Family Nurse Practitioner Review and Resource Manual, 4th Edition* as a supplement for greater detail on the non-clinical subjects and the clinical subjects I had trouble grasping.

Besides using Fitzgerald's certification review book, I took a certification review course soon after graduation, again Fitzgerald. I'm by no means advocating that you should use Fitzgerald for your review materials, I just liked her style in regards to the information presented. Browse through a few books yourself and decide what works best for you. I enjoyed my review class, and it was a great help to put things together that I didn't quite grasp in school. Because of this, I advise senior NP students to take a review course while they are still in school.

My review course was over a weekend and cost a few hundred dollars. I actually coordinated the event and had a review instructor come to teach the course for our school. You can do this by contacting the specific review course you are interested in and ask if they would be willing to host a class for a group of you and your classmates.

The company wants to make sure you have a certain number of people interested before they will even consider coming out to you. If enough of your classmates are interested, they will come to your area and host a class on a date that is convenient for you. This was a great deal considering that travel and accommodations could add up to the thousands depending on where you're going.

I gave myself one full month to study after I received the authorization to test (ATT) from ANCC. I wanted to get completely through my review book and feel confident I was familiar with concepts that could be on the exam.

During this time I also purchased some practice exams from www.familynpprep.com and took two practice exams per week that month. This site allows you the opportunity to review the questions you get wrong after the exam, and I made the most of that feature. I made flashcards from the questions I answered incorrectly so that I could take them with me to work and study on my downtime.

This method was my basic study technique for the exam, here it is in list format:

- Purchase a review book during last semester of school and study for school exams with it.

- Take a review course during the last few weeks of class or right after school.

- Read your review book from front to back and answer all practice questions. Make a schedule of what you will study and when, coordinating it with your work schedule (I usually did my online tests on the days I worked).

- If you have a second, more detailed, review book read over the subject for the day to re-enforce your subject. (i.e. Hematology in Fitzgerald's book, Read and review in ANCC review book)

- Get a supplemental review book if needed to clarify information or go into greater detail of subjects where you're having trouble.

- Take online practice tests, at least two per week, and make flashcards to study with during work.

- Study consistently, whenever and wherever you can until your testing date. Make sure you take off two days before the exam to give yourself time to relax before the big day.

Sample Study Calendar

Sunday	Monday	Tuesday	Wednesday	Thursday	Friday	Saturday
Off	Work 7a-7p Health Promotion & Disease prevention	Work 7a-7p Practice Exam	Neurology	Work 7a-7p Practice Exam	Skin Disorders	Psychosocial Disorders
Work 7a-7p	Eye, Ears, Nose, Throat	Cardiology	Work 7a-7p Practice exam	Work 7a-7p Gerontology	Practice Exam	Female Reproductive and GU systems
Off	Abdominal Disorders	Work 7a-7p Practice Exam	Work 7a-7p Male GU	Musculoskeletal Practice Exam	Work 7a-7p Peripheral Vascular Disease	Pediatrics
Off	Work 7a-7p Practice Exam	Work 7a-7p	Endocrine	Work 7a-7p Practice Exam	Hematological and Immunological Disorders	Childbearing
Work 7a-7p Practice Exam	Work 7a-7p	Work 7a-7p Practice Exam	Off	Off	Test Day	

Nurse Practitioner Certification Boards Contact Information

American Nurses Credentialing Center
8515 Georgia Avenue, Suite 400
Silver Spring, MD 20910-3492
Phone: 1-800-284-2378

American Association of Nurse Practitioners
P.O. Box 12846
Austin, TX 78711
Phone: (512) 442-4262
Fax: (512) 442-6469
admin@aanp.org

National Certification Corporation
676 N. Michigan Ave, Suite 3600
Chicago, IL 60611
Phone: 312-951-0207
info@nccnet.org

Pediatric Nursing Certification Board
9605 Medical Center Drive, Suite 250
Rockville, Maryland 20850
Phone: (301) 330-2921
Toll Free: 1-888-641-2767
Fax: 301-330-1504

Chapter 8
Landing Your First Job

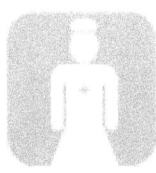

As a student approaching graduation, you should get your resume ready to go. During your last semester of school you should put together a portfolio that will help you be more organized for when you do get your first job and any other job thereafter. Most of this you won't have until you land your first job, but get your folder organized early and add to it when you get these documents. Buy a 1-inch 3-ring binder with dividers and clear plastic pockets and include these items:

- Official transcripts
- Updated resume
- CME credits
- BLS/ACLS certifications
- Immunization records
- Copy of DEA number
- Copies of RN and APRN licenses
- Copies of NPI number
- Copies of malpractice insurance

- Certificates showing membership to professional organizations
- List and contact information of professional references

Having all of these documents together in a binder will help you with the credentialing process at every company where you work that receives insurance payments. Having these documents ready will save you time, as well as having them available on a scanning app on your phone.

Employers will love how fast you can get them required documents if you have your stuff together. You don't want to delay the credentialing process longer than necessary because of missing or lost documents. The longer the credentialing process, the less you get paid!

Bigger companies have a dedicated credentialing team who does a majority of the work for you by filling out the paperwork and just having you provide required documentation and signatures. Simple. But if you're working with a smaller company, more of them expect you to fill out the 20-pages of paperwork and everything else that entails. I've worked with both types of companies, and trust me – having someone automate the credentialing is so much easier.

The NP job market is tough in some geographical areas of the country, so it's best to start your job search while in the last few months of school. This is best accomplished by networking with other NPs and MDs with whom you work. Let all your associates know you will be graduating soon, and you are looking for a job.

I wish I had started looking for a job while I was in school instead of waiting until I took my boards two months later. It takes much more to get a job as an NP than any nursing job I've had. Many employers want you to do multiple interviews before they consider you for a position. Then you have to go through extensive credentialing for the insurance companies you will be billing.

Applying blindly to positions rarely works when you are a student who hasn't taken and passed their boards yet. This is why it is important to network, network, network. During your clinical rotations ask if openings are available at your clinical site or if your preceptors have any inside information on jobs. Another great way to network and find jobs is through your local NP association. Attend the meetings as often as you can as a student and remember to network at every possible opportunity.

If you are like me and waited until you passed your board exam, you can continue to apply for jobs during this time, but make sure you're still working or have adequate savings. It took me roughly 4 months to start my full-time NP job after going through the interviewing and credentialing process. Four months is actually fast for most geographical locations. I've heard of NPs not landing their first job for six months or longer. Imagine how much longer that is with a lengthy credentialing process!

Besides continuing to network, upload your resume on to the major job boards like Indeed and Zip Recruiter. Google "NP jobs" and find niche specific job boards where you can post your resume instead of a general job board. If you have a LinkedIn profile, update that as well. You never know who's looking at your profile and may be hiring.

A word on resumes...

Co-workers and friends always wanted me to review their resumes for them, and I found that many nurses do not know how to write a resume! Don't let your poor resume writing skills follow you into your new career as an NP.

First, make sure your grammar and punctuation are correct. If the person reviewing your resume was anything like me when I was a hiring manager, I'd toss it without a second glance, no matter how stellar your experience was. Second, keep your resume as succinct as possible by using action words and statements that get to the point. Excess words are not your friend here because hiring managers seldom read past your header before they decide they like you as a potential candidate. Format your resume to make it visually appealing. I don't mean by using fancy script fonts that the average person can't read. I mean by highlighting your strengths and accomplishments.

As far as your experience is concerned, do you list your clinical sites or not on a new grad NP resume? I didn't, and I received compliments on my resume all the time by people who were interested in hiring me. If someone is considering hiring me, they should know my scope of practice as an APRN. There's no need for me to waste precious resume space on clinical rotations. If they have questions about my experience, I clarify it in my interview. Be leery of potential employers who aren't aware of your full scope of competence or you may be expected to function as an RN. Something your resume *should* have though are bulleted points highlighting your experience.

Example:
- Suturing
- X-Ray interpretation
- Family Medicine

You get the point. Employers like looking at bullet points since they're easier to read than one big blob of words. Make your resume visually appealing through formatting. Words on a page are boring until you break things up with sections, headers, and bullet points. If you have an extensive work experience, you must correctly format it on a resume. I know many nurses have an extensive nursing background. Formatting can help you avoid looking like you're a job-hopper.

I made a few mistakes with my first job, and I want to help others avoid those mistakes early in my career. When you're new, you may apply to every NP opening you see without thinking how you would react if you got the job. Be picky about the ones where you spend time applying. You don't want to waste precious time when you could do something more productive.

5 Tips to Maximize Your Job Hunting Experience

1. Only apply for jobs where you are qualified. Don't spin your wheels, wasting time better spent doing something else. If you are an FNP, don't apply to an ACNP position and get mad when you don't get the job. Likewise, if recruiters contact you for jobs, immediately tell them your population focus and cut them off if they have offers for other than the capacity where you can work. I spent endless hours on the phone with people who talked up a

position only to find out I wasn't qualified because I was an FNP (because once again, they went off my previous RN experience).

2. Filter out recruiters who contact you. Recruiters were never useful for me until I was laid-off [5] for the second time and knew how to make them work for me. Recruiters who just randomly called and "wanted to talk" were always annoying to me. They would ask me about myself and what kind of job I wanted, but they had nothing to offer me. Finally, I started to cut the "talkers" off and pointedly told them, "If you don't have any specific job to present to me, I'm not interested in talking." This stopped a lot of them from randomly calling and fishing for information when they had nothing to offer. I only solicited recruiters who had offers for me. You should too.

3. Be open to other possibilities, but don't settle. Be open to other job opportunities that may come your way. You may have had your heart set on working in a community health clinic, but an opening for an internal medicine group becomes available. Although this is a completely different setting, as your first NP job you will gain knowledge that will serve you well in the future. My first NP job was a per-diem job that involved

going to patients' places of employment and conducting wellness assessments and education. I wasn't diagnosing or prescribing with that job, but the experience served me well in other positions I've had since then. The skill-set I gained from that position has helped me land jobs in health and wellness and occupational health. I also acquired some additional skills conducting the assessments online when the company changed to a telehealth model.

4. Use social media to your advantage. Clean up your social media pages if you have any questionable pictures, posts, or tweets. More and more employers are looking at applicant's social media pages to see if the person has any behavior that would damage their company. Get a LinkedIn account. If you don't already have one, upload your resume and update your profile. I still get offers on LinkedIn for jobs in my area. Reach out to your medical and nursing friends on Facebook to see if anyone has the inside scoop on positions in their company. Use Twitter to follow companies in which you are most interested and keep tabs if they tweet openings. They're likely to be impressed if you follow them already and then respond.

5. Keep a running list of the jobs for which you have applied. Then, you can contact them within two weeks after applying to avoid your resume getting lost on someone's desk. Another good reason to keep a list of jobs where you have applied is so you don't forget! On several occasions, someone has called me about a job to which I had applied, but they had to remind me of the position. You can avoid this embarrassment if you keep a list of jobs where you have applied and any pertinent information about the company.

The Interview

Congratulations, all your hard work has paid off, and you've got an interview coming! All the prepping you've done has paid off, but there's more you must do to land the job you want. Since you have graduated in a particular population focus, you should know the kind of job you want and can be choosy about potential job offers.

The key to landing a good job where you're valued as a provider and not exploited is to not be desperate and not jump on the first job offer you receive – unless it's a good deal of course. Rarely do newly graduated NPs find a perfect first job. Instead, they jump on the first offer and end up regretting it later when they realize they're working for peanuts or are still expected to function in a nurse role instead of as a provider.

If you dress appropriately, it will help you make a good first impression to the person who is interviewing you. Both men and women should wear business suits, with nice polished shoes and minimal accessories. Women should steer more on the conservative side with makeup and both sexes shouldn't douse themselves with perfume or cologne since many people have allergies. You don't want your interviewer allergic to you. That could create a bad first impression that ends the interview before it even begins!

Tips for Acing Your Interview

1. Dress for success

2. Perfect Your Body Language

3. Practice interviewing

4. Be prepared for odd questions

5. Research the company

6. Be on-time

7. Follow-up with a "Thank you" note

Perfect your Body Language

Your overall body language can send vibes that turn off an interviewer. Enter the room with confidence by standing up straight and no slouching, offering a firm handshake, and waiting to be seated until told so. You probably already know this, but gum and mints during the interview are a no-no. Make sure you discard them before you walk into the place where you are meeting your potential employer.

Practice Interviewing

If you're not experienced at interviewing, take time to practice before your big day. Review some of the most common questions and practice your response in a mirror or with a friend. The interview will go by more smoothly if you are prepared for the most common questions asked like "What is your greatest strength?" "What is your greatest weakness?" "If you could change something about yourself, what would it be?"

Be Prepared for Odd Questions

If you prepare for the common questions, you're also going to have to prepare for the odd ones. There will be some questions that throw you a curve ball. Hopefully by the time you get to them in your interview, you will have had time to think through them without wasting precious brainpower on the easy ones. When presented with an odd interview question, think though it before answering. Sometimes interviewers ask these questions just to see how you think on your feet.

Research the Company

Do your research on any company where you are interviewing before the interview. Google them and check out their Facebook, Twitter and LinkedIn page. Doing this will give you key information about the company before you enter the room and plenty of talking points during the interview. Doing this not only allows you to know more about the company for your own personal knowledge, but it impresses your interviewer at the same time. It's great to know to know the company's values and missions and work it into your interview.

Be on Time

For any interview you have, be on time! Tardiness for an employment interview is a big turn-off for any interviewer. Do a test drive to the interview site the day before your meeting and time when you leave so you won't arrive late. Consider traffic if you live in a major city. Plan to arrive 10-15 minutes before your scheduled interview time.

Follow-up with a Thank You Note

Always thank the interviewer for taking the time to interview you. You can do this one of two ways: via email or snail mail. In our time, many people are connected to their email, and I've found great success sending out an email later on the same day after an interview. Usually interviewers will give you a business card and ask you to follow-up if you have any other questions not covered during the interview. Use the contact information to send a Thank You card after your interview. The only problem is the possibility that the card will be misplaced or the recipient might not open it in time to improve your chances to get the job.

Questions You Need to Ask During an Interview

Now that you have the basics of the interview in order, it is time to review what to expect from your NP interview. Your main job during the interview is to listen with a third ear and even take notes if you feel the need. You want to be 100% sure what is expected of you.

Usually the interviewers will give a lot of voluntary information in the beginning because they've interviewed dozens before you and want to get to the point. It's good if the interviewer gives you a detailed description of the job for which you're interviewing. I've been to interviews where I felt like I was pulling teeth to get details on the job.

The person doing the interview should be willing to answer any questions you have about the job. Employers are usually happy to answer questions and are impressed by candidates who ask meaningful questions during the interview. As an NP, you should ask many questions to clarify that your role is different than it was as an RN. Many of these questions involve the benefits package. Don't be afraid of asking them upfront. You need to know this information to make an informed decision if you are offered the position.

Here are some key questions you need to ask on any interview you participate in:

1. How am I paid (salary, hourly, revenue, salary + revenue)?

2. What are my expected hours and days to work?

3. Is call required, if so, how often, and at what rate?

4. Do you offer benefits and what benefits do you offer?

    a. Medical
    b. Dental

c. Vision
   d. 401k (with or without employee matching?)
   e. Short-term and Long-term disability
   f. Malpractice (occurrence or claims-made?)
   g. Do you cover licensure renewal and DEA fees?
   h. Vacation (how many days)
   1. Continuing medical education (CME) (How many days and how much money?)

5. Are relocation expenses paid?

6. Is there a sign-on bonus?

7. Will I be able to go over my revenue for the company with the biller?

8. Does the company offer any quarterly or yearly bonus?

9. Does the company have yearly raises?

10. Has this company ever had an NP work for them before?

11. Has anyone here ever worked with an NP before?

12. If this isn't a new position, why did the last person leave?

13. Do you offer an orientation period and if so, how long is it?

14. Who do I report to regarding medical, administrative, and billing concerns?

15. Is the NP required to supervise any of the office support staff?

16. When do you expect to make a hiring decision?

Questions You Will Probably be Asked During an Interview

There will be the standard questions like, "What is your greatest strength or weakness?" but be prepared to answer questions about what you, as an NP, can bring to the practice. Most interviewers want to know why they should hire you (especially if you're a new grad) instead of John Doe they interviewed yesterday.

This situation is especially true if the company where you are interviewing has little or no experience working with an NP.

You should be prepared to answer these questions:

1. What is your skill-set as a (blank—Your specialty here) NP?
2. Can you practice independently?

3. How many patients are you accustomed to seeing per day?
4. Do you have a DEA number?
5. What can you legally do?
6. Can you work weekends, evenings, and holidays?
7. How do you feel about being the only provider in the clinic?
8. Can you float between clinics?

I was offered a job, now what?

First, congratulations on the job offer! Now is the time for you to evaluate the offer and negotiate if needed. Weigh your options carefully, and make sure you have all the needed information before you accept an offer, counter their offer, or reject it.

Make sure they offer the job and its terms in writing. Nothing can be done later if your employer is doing something not specified in the contract when you first started. As an NP, you should expect some industry standard benefits in addition to your base salary to be covered. The amount covered varies by employer, but the consensus between most NPs is that in addition to making no less than $100,000 as a base salary you should be provided the following benefits.

- Malpractice insurance
- CME $1,000-$1,500

- CME days (5)
- Vacation (3 weeks)
- Medical/Dental/Vision insurance
- Short and Long term disability insurance
- Coverage of all licenses, registration, and DEA fees

If you need to negotiate your offer, do so even if it may make you feel uncomfortable. It never hurts to ask, and you'll regret it if you didn't and you could have made an additional $5,000 a year. A study in the *Journal of Organizational Behavior*[6] estimates you could lose over $600,000 in salary during a typical career. That's a lot of money! The absolute minimum you should accept is a $100k base salary. I cannot stress this enough. I hear so many NPs tell me they took a job earning less than the national average because they don't have experience, or that they were tired of looking and took the first job offered. Please do not do this! It makes things harder for all NPs when any NP takes a job for less than what we are worth.

If this is your first NP job, you must display confidence in your abilities and believe you are worth the national average. If you have any NP experience, focus on the value you will bring to the company, and ask for at least 10% more if they try to low-ball you with their offer.

You will usually be communicating with a recruiter or Human Resources instead of the person who interviewed you. In my opinion, this makes it easier to negotiate since a third party is involved. Be prepared to walk away if you don't come to an agreement that works for you. Remember to get everything in writing after all salary and benefit negotiations are done.

Negotiating skills take some practice to develop and some confidence to carry out. Read on the subject so you will feel more comfortable during the job-hunting process.

Chapter 9
Life After School

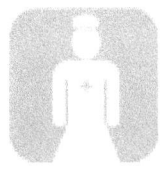

Right after I graduated, I had many questions about what I was supposed to do next after taking my board exam. I knew there were official numbers I needed to obtain, but I didn't know the sequencing of how to get them. Was I supposed to get my DPS, then my DEA, or did I get them at the same time? What did I need to get to prescribe non-scheduled meds? What is an NPI number?

You see, some NP schools leave a lot for graduates to figure out on their own. We had one class toward the end of the year (for one hour) that covered these important topics, but it was too much for such a short time to digest. From what I've heard from other NP colleagues, they also had problems obtaining this basic information in their programs.

There are five requirements that make you a legit NP ready to practice. Note that completion of these five steps does not necessarily allow you to prescribe medication, though. These requirements are for today's NP graduates. Years ago, a master's degree was not needed to become an NP. These NPs have since been grandfathered into practice and the below requirements do not apply to them.

Basic requirements for NP practice:
- Bachelor's degree in Nursing
- Registered Nurse License
- Graduate Nurse Education
- National Board Certification
- State NP licensure and/or registration (AANP infographic, 2016)[7]

Remember, state-required qualifications vary widely for NP practice. Currently, master's degrees are required in 34 states, and 45 states that require NPs to pass a national certification exam. There are also states that do not require NPs to pass a national certification exam. Check with your state's board of nursing for specifics.

Prescriptive Authority as an NP

There are additional requirements you may need to practice and prescribe as an NP, again depending on your state.

- National Provider Identification number (NPI)

- Prescriptive authority (if required by your state)
- Collaboration agreement (if in non-independent state)
- Drug Enforcement Administration number (DEA)

There will be slight variations in the process of obtaining these numbers depending on the state where you will be practicing and what you will need in terms of practice. For example, I didn't need a DEA for this first year of practice since I was in a specialty where scheduled drugs were not prescribed. I only needed prescriptive authority from the state of Texas.

NPs have the ability to prescribe in all 50 states and D.C. Each state has different requirements to obtain the right to prescribe. In the state of Texas, in addition to applying for your advanced practitioner recognition (license), you have the option to apply for prescriptive authority for an additional fee.

The prescriptive authority only gives you the authority to prescribe non-scheduled meds (non-narcotic). If you need to prescribe scheduled meds in your practice, you must obtain a DEA number. Again, the process is different in each state. Your state nursing board will provide details of what you need in your particular area.

*In Texas you needed a DPS number before you could be issued a DEA number. The rules have since changed, and as of September 1, 2016, a DPS number is no longer needed in Texas. Before you can get either number, if you work in a state that requires physician collaboration, you and the physician with whom you are working must fill out a collaboration agreement. In Texas it's a simple process where the NP enters their information on the Medical Board website and the physician approves the collaboration. Once the collaboration is finalized, the DEA number can be issued.

NPI number

The NPI number is a National Provider Identifier number required of all providers for billing purposes. It is a unique 10-digit number assigned to you by the federal government. Applying to get an NPI number is an easy process. You simply need to go to the NPI database and register. It took me one weekend to get this number. You don't even need to have a job to get this number. You can apply to this number at anytime, but as a word of warning, you will have to enter in an address. If you register with your home address, it will be visible to anyone who looks up your NPI for any reason. Get your NPI number here.[8]

Prescriptive Authority

Depending on your state, you may or may not need prescriptive authority through your nursing board. I just had to check a box and pay an extra fee, and it's renewed every time I renew my advanced practice license. Prescriptive authority is good for as long as you are licensed as an advanced practice nurse; meaning you renew it when you renew your license. In some states the prescriptive authority is granted at the time of advanced practice licensure, in others, you have to apply separately. Prescriptive authority only allows you to prescribe non-scheduled medication.

Collaboration Agreement

The collaboration agreement with a physician may or may not be needed in your state. Check your nursing board to see if you have this requirement. Each state has different requirements for how often a physician should meet with an NP and for how long. Specific state requirements for you state can be found here.[9]

DEA number

A DEA number allows you to prescribe scheduled drugs. This is a federally provided number, for which you can submit your application after any state-required licenses are obtained. Get your DEA number here.[10]

Try to negotiate your DEA number into your employment agreement since it is so costly (currently $731 for a 3-year registration). Good employers will cover the cost for their providers. You will need to be employed to obtain this number. It took me less than a month to get my number.

Classification of Controlled Substances

- *Schedule I*: No accepted medical use in the United States and have high abuse potential. Examples include heroin, LSD, and cocaine.

- *Schedule II*: Have a high abuse potential with severe psychic or physical dependence liability and generally are substances that have therapeutic utility. Examples include morphine, hydrocodone, methadone, and fentanyl.

- *Schedule III*: Are stimulants and depressants with an abuse potential that is less than those drugs in Schedules I and II. Examples include mixtures of limited specified quantities of codeine with noncontrolled active ingredients (such as Tylenol #3) and mixtures of amobarbital, pentobarbital, or secobarbital with other noncontrolled medicinal ingredients.

- *Schedule IV*: These drugs have less abuse potential than Schedule III and include depressants such as alprazolam, phenobarbital, and chloral hydrate.

- *Schedule V*: These substances have less abuse potential than Schedule IV and include preparations containing limited quantities of certain narcotic and stimulant drugs generally given for antitussive, antidiarrheal, and analgesic purposes. Examples include buprenorphine and propylhexedrin. (Buppert, 2015) [11]

Prescription Writing

You'll be doing a lot of prescription writing in and out of school, and when you start it can be kind of tricky. Most practices have gone to EMR (electric medical records), so you may never actually have to write out a prescription on a prescription pad, but you will need to know how for school.

Surprisingly, I don't recall anyone going over the basics of prescription-writing in school, and it was something I picked up during clinicals with my first preceptor. It's not hard, but there are required aspects you need to include so the pharmacist doesn't call you for clarification when the patient goes to pick up their prescription.

Here is what you need to include on each prescription:

Patient Name: This is a no-brainer, but it's the most basic of writing a prescription. Don't forget to write your patients name on the prescription.

Patients D.O.B.: This patient identifier is commonly included on prescriptions along with patient's addresses sometimes depending on where you work. This is to make sure that the prescription is going to the correct person.

Medication Name: Next up is the medication you want to prescribe. It doesn't matter if you write the brand name or generic name unless you specifically want the patient to take one or another. If you want to order the brand name, the bottom of the prescription should have a box on the bottom where you check that says "Do not Substitute" or "Substitutions not allowed."

- **Strength**: Here you write in the medication strength. Let's say you are prescribing Ibuprofen. Ibuprofen comes in many strengths, OTC and prescription. How much do you want to prescribe? 200mg, 400mg, 600mg or 800mg? This must be clarified on your prescription.

- **Amount**: Do you want your patient to take 1, 2, or 3 pills? Here is where you write the quantity of the medication you want the patient to take at one time.

- **Route**: Here you have to specify whether you want the patient to take the medication by mouth, sublingually, rectally or one of many other ways medication can be administered.

- **Frequency**: How often can the patient take the medication? Every 2,4, or 6 hours? Every day? Every other day?

Why: What is the reason the patient is taking the medication? You have to specify the reason you are prescribing the medication, is it as needed for pain, indigestion, or constipation?

How Much: This is where you tell the pharmacist how much of the medication to fill. Write out the quality in both numerical form and written form. Example: Dispense #30 (thirty).

Refills: Are you going to allow your patient to have refills, if so, how many?

Here's a great resource for writing prescriptions.[12] Apparently, medical students don't get much covered in school either.

What Exactly do I Need to Keep up With as an NP?

If you're an NP who has prescriptive authority and work in a collaborating state this is what you will need to keep track of:

- Registered Nurse License (renewed every 1-4 years, depending on state)
- Advanced Practice Nurse License/ Registration (same as RN renewal)
- Board Certification (Every 1-5 years depending on certification)
- Prescriptive authority (same as RN renewal)
- Other state-specific licensure (varies)
- DEA (every 3 years)
- Continuing Education (same as RN renewal)

There is a lot to keep track of, so again, use a 3-ring binder to store all this information and use reminders in your personal calendar to keep up. Your employer may also remind you of upcoming renewal dates, but don't count on this. Keep up with your own certifications so you won't have to involuntary stop working because one of your licenses or registration has lapsed.

An NP, by any Other Name

The term Nurse Practitioner is a generic term for our profession, but did you know that each state has different titles for NPs? Depending on what state you live in you could be known as an APN, APRN, CRNP, or just NP. Let's take a look at the official titles for NPs in each state.

Alabama: Certified Registered Nurse Practitioner (CRNP)

Alaska: Advanced Nurse Practitioner (ANP)

Arizona: Registered Nurse Practitioner (RNP)

Arkansas: Registered Nurse Practitioner (RNP)

California: Nurse Practitioner (NP)

Colorado: Nurse Practitioner (NP)

Connecticut: Advanced Practice Registered Nurse (APRN) or Certified Nurse Practitioner (CNP)

Delaware: Advanced Practice Nurse (APN), Advanced Registered Nurse Practitioner (ARNP)

or Nurse Practitioner (NP)

District of Columbia: Advanced Practice Registered Nurse (APRN)

Florida: Advanced Registered Nurse Practitioner (ARNP)

Georgia: Advanced Practice Registered Nurse (APRN) or Nurse Practitioner (NP)

Hawaii: Advanced Practice Registered Nurse (APRN)

Idaho: Advanced Practice Registered Nurse (APRN)

Illinois: Advanced Practice Nurse (APN)

Indiana: Advanced Practice Nurse (APN) or Nurse Practitioner (NP)

Iowa: Advanced Registered Nurse Practitioner (ARNP) or Certified Nurse Practitioner (CNP)

Kansas: Advanced Practice Registered Nurse (APRN)

Kentucky: Advanced Practice Registered Nurse (APRN)

Louisiana: Advanced Practice Registered Nurse (APRN)

Maine: Advanced Practice Registered Nurse (APRN) or Certified Nurse Practitioner (CNP)

Maryland: Certified Registered Nurse Practitioner (CRNP)

Massachusetts: Nurse Practitioner (NP)

Michigan: Certified Nurse Practitioner (CNP)

Minnesota: Advanced Practice Registered Nurse (APRN) or Nurse Practitioner (NP)

Mississippi: Advanced Practice Registered Nurse (APRN)

Missouri: Advanced Practice Registered Nurse (APRN)

Montana: Advanced Practice Registered Nurse (APRN) or Nurse Practitioner (NP)

Nebraska: Nurse Practitioner (NP)

Nevada: Advanced Practice Registered Nurse (APRN)

New Hampshire: Advanced Practice Registered Nurse (APRN)

New Jersey: Advanced Practice Nurse (APN)

New Mexico: Certified Nurse Practitioner (CNP)

New York: Nurse Practitioner (NP)

North Carolina: Advanced Practice Registered Nurse (APRN) or Nurse Practitioner (NP)

North Dakota: Advanced Practice Registered Nurse (APRN) or Nurse Practitioner (NP)

Ohio: Certified Nurse Practitioner (CNP) or Advanced Practice Registered Nurse (APRN)

Oklahoma: Advanced Practice Nurse (APN) or Advanced Registered Nurse Practitioner (ARNP)

Oregon: Nurse Practitioner (NP)

Pennsylvania: Certified Registered Nurse Practitioner (CRNP)

Rhode Island: Certified Registered Nurse Practitioner (CRNP)

South Carolina: Nurse Practitioner (NP)

South Dakota: Nurse Practitioner (NP)

Tennessee: Advanced Practice Nurse (APN) or Certified Nurse Practitioner (CNP)

Texas: Advanced Practice Nurse (APN)

Utah: Advanced Practice Registered Nurse (APRN)

Vermont: Advanced Practice Registered Nurse (APRN)

Virginia: Nurse Practitioner (NP)

Washington: Advanced Registered Nurse Practitioner (ARNP)

West Virginia: Advanced Nurse Practitioner (ANP) or Nurse Practitioner (NP)

Wisconsin: Nurse Practitioner (NP)

Wyoming: Advanced Practice Registered Nurse (APRN)

(Buppert, 2015)[13]

How Do I Sign My Name Now That I'm an NP?

One pet peeve of mine is when I see NPs sign their names incorrectly. I see this all the time:

Jane Doe, RN, MSN, FNP, and it makes me cringe! As an NP there is no need to include the RN designation in your title, you must be an RN to be an NP, so leave it out.

Another thing I see all the time is the endless list of titles also known as alphabet soup: Jane Doe, MSN, BS, RN, APRN, FAAN, CCRN, FNP-BC. There is no need to list that many titles after your name. I know you earned them, and you are proud, but do you see MDs with an alphabet behind their name? I don't know if it's a complex issue or what, but you'll just end up confusing your patients and looking like you have an inferiority complex or something. Only sign what is necessary for your state and professional designation.

There are six basic type of credentials that you may have earned that can legally be used after your name listed by the least likely to be revoked.

Degree: These designations cannot be taken away, so list them first. They include your nursing degrees (ADN, BSN, MSN, PhD, DNP). They also include your non-nursing degrees (JD, MS, EdD). Please do not use every degree you have, if you have multiple degrees in nursing like I do, use the highest. If not, my signature would look like this: Nachole Johnson, CNA, LPN, ADN, BSN, MSN, RN, FNP-BC. If you have a nursing degree and a non-nursing degree, use your highest nursing degree and your highest non-nursing degree next. Example: Jane Doe, MSN, MPH, RN.

Licensure: These are awarded on the basis of your completed education and passing a national licensure exam (e.g., LPN, RN).

State designation or requirement: Each state is different in how it recognizes NPs. (See the section "*An NP by any Other Name*" for state NP designations). These credentials are authorized by each state based on completion of advanced education, or certain types of experience.

National Certification: These certification titles are awarded by the ANCC, AANP or other certifying body with whom you took your nurse practitioner boards. They give you the designation "C" with AANP or "BC" with ANCC (using the two most common examples).

Awards or honors: These are given when individuals are recognized for their outstanding service or accomplishments. Examples are FAAN (Fellow of the American Academy of Nursing) and the FCCM (Fellow of Critical Care Medicine).

Other Certifications: These can include a wide variety of certifications that indicate additional skills acquired through education or testing like CCRN.

By taking all this into account, I would sign my name as Nachole Johnson, MSN, APN, FNP-BC. This is a lot simpler to read, don't you agree?[14]

One Last Thing

Getting into NP school, graduating, passing boards, and landing your first job can be a daunting experience. I hope I was able to clarify some of the questions you had before you started the book. If you enjoyed this book and learned something insightful, please share by leaving a review on my Amazon page amazon.com/author/nacholejohnson While you're there be sure to check out my other books that will help in your career as an NP.

About the Author

Nachole Johnson is a nurse practitioner who loves educating and inspiring other nurses to succeed in life. She has authored numerous blogs and articles for Minority Nurse Magazine and Dailynurse.com .She is also the author of multiple books including *You're a Nurse and Want to Start Your Own Business? The Complete Guide.* In addition, she is founder of Renursing Career Consulting, a company dedicated to empowering nurses. Learn more at amazon.com/author/nacholejohnson

Other Books By Nachole Johnson

You're a Nurse and Want to Start Your Own Business? The Complete Guide

50+ Business Ideas for the Entrepreneurial Nurse

Notes

[1] http://www.medscape.com/viewarticle/810692 and http://bmchealthservres.biomedcentral.com/articles/10.1186/1472-6963-14-214

[2] BMC Health Serv Res. 2014 May 12;14:214. doi: 10.1186/1472-6963-14-214.
Substitution of physicians by nurses in primary care: a systematic review and meta-analysis.
Martínez-González NA, Djalali S, Tandjung R, Huber-Geismann F, Markun S, Wensing M, Rosemann T1.

[3] www.apna.org, www.vanderbilt.edu , www.pncb.org

[4] http://www.thestudygurus.com

[5] See my book [The Financially Savvy NP: Your Guide to Building Wealth] which tells more about this experience and how you can avoid such situations in your career.

[6] http://lifehacker.com/5968375/not-negotiating-your-starting-salary-could-cost-you-500000

[7] https://www.aanp.org/images/about-nps/npgraphic.pdf

[8] https://nppes.cms.hhs.gov/NPPES/Welcome.do

[9] https://www.aanp.org/legislation-regulation/state-legislation/state-practice-environment

[10] https://www.deadiversion.usdoj.gov/

[11] Buppert, Carolyn. Nurse Practitioner's Business Practice And Legal Guide. Jones & Bartlett Learning: 5th Edition (May 15, 2014), 199-204.

[12] http://medicalschoolhq.net/prescription-writing-101/

[13] Buppert. *Nurse Practitioner's Business.* Appendix 1-A.

[14] http://nursingworld.org/FunctionalMenuCategories/Abo

utANA/Leadership-Governance/NewCNPE/CNPEMembersOnly/CNPEReferenceDocuments/PlayingtheCredentialsGame.pdf

www.ingramcontent.com/pod-product-compliance
Lightning Source LLC
Chambersburg PA
CBHW060404190526
45169CB00002B/747